TITLE PAGE

REMAIN
FIT
FOR
LIFE

Your Ultimate Guide
to
Staying Healthy and Active

DISCLAIMER

TABLE OF CONTENTS

book review

 Fit for Life is an outstanding aide that enables perusers to assume command over their well-being and settle on informed conclusions about their prosperity. Its comprehensive methodology, upheld by logical proof, separates it from other eating regimens and nourishment books. Whether you're looking for weight reduction, expanded energy, or a total way of life update, Fit for Life offers an abundance of significant data to show you the way to a better, more energetic life.

about the author

Prof Paul.k.chesley is a first-in-class maker and teacher, an exceptional event speaker, and an essayist. In over 10 years working with Ramsey

Courses of Action, he has conveyed his certain message to swarms across the world appearance vast people how to expect control over their assets and achieve their objectives. and how to find actual success throughout everyday life book audit

Presentation:

Welcome to "Fit Forever: Your Definitive Manual for Remaining Sound and Dynamic." In our current reality where our ways of life have become progressively stationary and our time is loaded up with furious timetables, it's a higher priority than at any other time to focus on our actual prosperity. This exhaustive aide expects to furnish you with the information and devices important to roll out sure improvements in your day-to-day existence and leave you on an excursion towards ideal well-being and essentialness.

In this quick-moving current period, tracking down the right harmony between work, family, and individual responsibilities can be a steady test. Frequently, our own well-being assumes a lower priority as we focus on different obligations. Nonetheless, keeping a fit and solid way of life isn't just about looking great yet additionally about feeling better, both genuinely and intellectually.

"Fit Forever" is intended to engage you with down-to-earth methodologies, master counsel, and noteworthy hints to assist you with integrating activity, sustenance, and care into your day-to-day everyday practice. Whether you're a novice beginning your wellness process or somebody hoping to take their ongoing wellness level higher than ever, this guide has something for everybody.

All through this aid, we will investigate different parts of remaining fit, including compelling exercise routine schedules, the significance of a reasonable eating regimen, systems for remaining spurred, and procedures for overseeing pressure. We'll dig into the most recent examination and give proof-based data to assist you with settling on informed decisions about your well-being.

Keep in mind, wellness is certainly not a one-size-fits-all idea. We as a whole have exceptional bodies, objectives, and difficulties. That is the reason "Fit Forever" centers around fitting the counsel to suit individual requirements and inclinations. We'll assist you with finding exercises you appreciate, solid recipes that entice your taste buds, and commonsense strategies to beat hindrances that might hold you up.

Chapter 1

Welcome to Fit Forever

Key thought 1. accepting a Sound and Dynamic Way of Life

In our current reality where requests and obligations frequently consume our significant investment, focusing on our well-being and prosperity is essential. Embracing a solid and dynamic way of life isn't simply a pattern; it's a cognizant decision to put resources into ourselves and develop propensities that help our drawn-out physical and mental essentials.

At its center, embracing a solid and dynamic way of life implies settling on purposeful choices that advance in general well-being. It includes taking on good dieting propensities, participating in standard actual work, and sustaining our psychological and profound prosperity. By finding a way proactive ways to really focus on ourselves, we can upgrade our personal satisfaction and open our maximum capacity.

One of the vital mainstays of a sound and dynamic way of life is nourishment. Filling our bodies with healthy, supplement-thick food sources gives the fundamental structure blocks to ideal working. It's tied in with consolidating a fair eating regimen wealthy in natural products, vegetables, entire grains, lean proteins, and solid fats. By feeding ourselves with the right supplements, we can uphold our invulnerable framework, keep a solid weight, and decrease the gamble of persistent sicknesses.

Actual work is one more fundamental part of a sound way of life. Taking part in customary activity works on our actual wellness as well as lifts our mindset, builds our energy levels, and upgrades our mental capability. It can take different structures, from cardiovascular exercises like running or cycling to strength preparation, yoga, or group activities. Finding exercises we appreciate guarantees that exercise turns into an economical piece of our daily practice.

Similarly significant is focusing on our psychological and profound prosperity. Embracing care rehearses, like contemplation, profound breathing activities, or journaling, can assist us with overseeing pressure, improving mindfulness, and developing a positive outlook. Getting some margin for taking care of oneself, defining limits, and encouraging sound connections all add to our by and large mental prosperity.

Embracing a solid and dynamic way of life isn't about flawlessness or unbending principles; about finding equilibrium and pursuing manageable decisions that line up with our singular requirements and values. It's tied in with being thoughtful of ourselves, embracing progress over flawlessness, and perceiving that little strides toward positive change can yield huge long-haul benefits.

All through this aid, we will investigate reasonable systems, master counsel, and motivation to assist you with accepting a sound and dynamic way of life.

From tips on dinner arranging and wellness schedules to care procedures and taking care of oneself practices, we'll give the apparatuses you want to roll out enduring improvements. Together, how about we set out on this groundbreaking excursion, where taking care of oneself and personal development become vital pieces of our regular routines? Prepare to focus on your well-being, raise your prosperity, and experience the significant prizes that accompany embracing a solid and dynamic way of life.

Key thought 2

The Significance of Focusing on Your Prosperity.

In the high-speed and requesting world, we live in, disregarding our own prosperity while shuffling endless responsibilities is simple. In any case, focusing on your prosperity isn't simply an extravagance or a bit of hindsight — it's an essential need for a satisfying and healthy lifestyle.

At its center, focusing on your prosperity implies perceiving that your physical, mental, and close-to-home well-being are the establishment whereupon all the other things are constructed. At the point when you deal with yourself, you're better prepared to deal with the difficulties and requests of day-to-day existence, and you can appear as the best version of yourself in all areas — work, connections, and special goals.

One of the key motivations behind why focusing on your prosperity is fundamental is its effect on your general well-being. At the point when you pursue cognizant decisions to focus on taking care of yourself, you're putting resources into your drawn-out actual prosperity. Ordinary activity, adjusted nourishment, and adequate rest are fundamental parts of a sound way of life. By participating in actual work, you reinforce your cardiovascular framework, work on your solidarity and adaptability, help your safe framework, and lessen the gamble of persistent illnesses. Dealing with your actual well-being improves your personal satisfaction presently as well as makes way for a better future.

Similarly significant is the effect of focusing on your psychological and profound prosperity. In a general public where stress, nervousness, and burnout are pervasive, effectively focusing on your emotional well-being becomes pivotal. Focusing on taking care of oneself exercises like care, contemplation, and unwinding procedures can assist with decreasing feelings of anxiety, further develop concentration and fixation, and upgrade your general close-to-home flexibility. At the point when you get some margin to support your psychological and close-to-home prosperity, you develop a feeling of inward harmony and dependability that emphatically impacts each part of your life.

Focusing on your prosperity likewise assumes a critical part in your connections and communications with others. At the point when you focus on taking care of yourself, you recharge your own energy savings, which permits you to be more present, compassionate, and steady toward people around you. It empowers you to lay out sound limits, impart actuality, and develop satisfying associations with others. By dealing with yourself, you become better prepared to deal with the necessities of others, cultivating better connections and a more agreeable public activity.

At last, focusing on your prosperity is a demonstration of self-confidence and self-esteem. It's tied in with perceiving your natural worth and recognizing that your requirements and bliss matter. By focusing on yourself, you send a strong message that you have the right to carry on with an existence of satisfaction, delight, and equilibrium.

In this aid, we will investigate different techniques and practices to assist you with focusing on your prosperity. From taking care of oneself customs and stressing the executive's methods to methodologies for balance between serious and fun activities and sustaining sound connections, we'll give you the instruments and information to focus on your prosperity. Keep in mind, by Section

chapter 2

Understanding Wellness:

Key thought 1 Defining Wellness and its Parts

Wellness is a wide idea that includes the general condition in great shape and sound. It goes past simple actual appearance and includes numerous parts that add to one's general wellness level. Understanding these parts can assist us in fostering a balanced way to deal with accomplishing and keeping up with ideal wellness. We should investigate the critical parts of wellness:

Cardiovascular Perseverance: Cardiovascular perseverance alludes to the capacity of the heart, veins, and lungs to supply oxygen and supplements to the functioning muscles during delayed active work productively. Frequently estimated by exercises hoist the pulse over a lengthy period, like running, swimming, cycling, or lively strolling. Further developing cardiovascular perseverance upgrades endurance, decreases the gamble of cardiovascular sicknesses, and supports by and large perseverance in everyday exercises.

Strong Strength: Solid strength alludes to the greatest power that a muscle or gathering of muscles can apply against the obstruction. It includes the capacity to produce power and beat obstruction, whether through bodyweight activities, weightlifting, or opposition preparation. Creating solid strength advances better stance, bone well-being, and practical strength for regular exercises.

Strong Perseverance: Solid perseverance is the capacity of muscles to support rehashed withdrawals over a drawn-out period without weakness. It centers around the ability to perform practices for a drawn-out term, for example, standing firm on a board situation or playing out various reiterations of an activity. Further developing strong perseverance adds to further developed execution in exercises that require supported muscle constrictions, like significant distance running or cycling.

Adaptability: Adaptability alludes to the scope of movement around a joint. It is impacted by the versatility of muscles, ligaments, and tendons. Normal extending activities, yoga, and portability work can further develop adaptability. Adaptability preparing upgrades joint versatility lessens the gamble of wounds, and further develops stance and general development quality.

Body Structure: The body piece alludes to the proportion of fat mass to incline mass in the body. It is a significant mark of generally speaking wellbeing and wellness. Accomplishing a sound body piece includes keeping a proper harmony between bulk and muscle-to-fat ratio. A balanced workout regime ought to mean diminishing the overabundance muscle to fat ratio while safeguarding or expanding fit bulk.

Equilibrium and Coordination: Equilibrium and coordination include the capacity to keep up with command over body developments and stance. Activities like yoga, kendo, and adjustment drills can further develop equilibrium and coordination. Upgrading these abilities diminishes the gamble of falls, further develops sports execution, and supports by and large development effectiveness.

Spryness and Speed: Deftness alludes to the capacity to head in a different path rapidly and effectively. Speed connects with the capacity to move quickly starting with one point and then onto the next. Dexterity and speed are fundamental for sports execution and can be upgraded through unambiguous preparation penetrates and works out.

Mental and Profound Prosperity: While not generally viewed as a part of wellness, mental and close-to-home prosperity are necessary to by and large wellness. Keeping up with great psychological well-being, overseeing pressure, and encouraging positive feelings add to a reasonable and solid way of life.

Understanding and integrating these parts of wellness into a balanced workout routine can assist you with accomplishing extensive wellness and working on your general well-being. It is vital to recollect that everybody's wellness level and objectives are exceptional, so it's crucial to plan a workout regime that suits your singular requirements and inclinations.

Key thought 2Assessing Your Ongoing Wellness Level

Surveying your ongoing wellness level is a significant stage in planning a compelling workout schedule and laying out reasonable objectives. It gives a benchmark estimation of your actual capacities and assists you with keeping tabs on your development after some time. Here are a few strategies and contemplations to survey your ongoing wellness level:

Self-Evaluation: Begin by thinking about your ongoing degree of actual work and by and large well-being. Consider factors, for example, your action level over the course of the day, any normal workout schedules you follow, and any medical issues or wounds that might influence your actual abilities. This self-evaluation gives an emotional comprehension of your wellness level and fills in as a beginning stage for development.

Oxygen-consuming Limit: Evaluating your high-impact limit gives experience in your cardiovascular perseverance. One normal technique is the "Talk Test" - on the off chance that you can keep a discussion while participating in moderate-force oxygen-consuming activity, your wellness level is probably normal. On the off chance that the discussion becomes troublesome, your wellness level might be lower. On the other hand, you can play out a wellness test, for example, a 1-mile walk/run or a stage test, to equitably gauge your high-impact wellness more.

Strength and Strong Perseverance: Assessing your solidarity and strong perseverance decides your ongoing degree of strong wellness. You can perform fundamental activities like push-ups, squats, or boards and note the number of reiterations or spans you can support. Contrasting your presentation with laid-out wellness benchmarks or age-and-orientation explicit standards can give bits of knowledge into your overall strength and solid perseverance.

Adaptability: Surveying your adaptability helps measure your scope of movement and joint portability. Basic tests like the sit-and-arrive at test or shoulder adaptability activities can give a general comprehension of your adaptability level. Focus on any constraints or uneasiness you experience during these tests.

Body Structure: Evaluating your body creation provides you with a comprehension of your overall measure of muscle-to-fat ratio and fit bulk. Techniques, for example, muscle versus fat calipers, bioelectrical impedance investigation, or double energy X-beam absorptiometry (DXA) outputs can give more exact estimations. On the other hand, visual appraisals and following changes in body estimations can likewise offer bits of knowledge into changes in body organization.

Practical Development Appraisal: Assessing your utilitarian development designs distinguishes any lopsided characteristics, shortcomings, or constraints in your development quality. Utilitarian development appraisals, like the squat, lurch, or single-leg balance tests, can give experiences into your capacity to perform essential developments actually and recognize regions for development.

It's vital to take note that wellness appraisals ought to be led with alertness, particularly assuming you have basic ailments or wounds. Consider talking with medical services proficient or ensured wellness master to direct you through the evaluation interaction and decipher the outcomes precisely.

By evaluating your ongoing wellness level, you can put forth practical objectives, plan a suitable workout schedule, and keep tabs on your development actually. Standard reassessment over the long run permits you to gauge upgrades and make fundamental changes in accordance with your daily schedule, guaranteeing proceeded with progress towards your ideal wellness results.

Key thought 3

Setting Reasonable Objectives for Progress

Laying out sensible objectives is pivotal for keeping up with inspiration, following advancement, and making long-haul progress in your wellness process. Ridiculous objectives can prompt dissatisfaction and frustration, while practical objectives give a make way and a feeling of achievement. Here are a few rules to assist you with laying out reasonable wellness objectives:

Be Explicit: Obviously, characterize your objectives. Rather than an obscure objective like "get fit," make it more unambiguous, for example, "shed 10 pounds" or "run a 5K race in less than 30 minutes." Explicit objectives give clearness and empower you to make an arrangement custom-made to your ideal result.

Make Them Quantifiable: Put forth objectives that can be estimated dispassionately. This permits you to keep tabs on your development and decide whether you're drawing nearer to your objective. Quantifiable objectives could incorporate practicing a specific number of days of the week, finishing a particular number of push-ups or squats, or lessening your mile show time to a particular sum.

Think about Your Beginning stage: Consider your ongoing wellness level and abilities. Defining objectives that are excessively difficult or requesting from the outset might prompt burnout or injury. Recognize your beginning stage and fabricate your objectives steadily to take into account continuous advancement.

Be Practical and Time-Bound: Put forth objectives that are feasible within a sensible time span. Think about elements like your way of life, responsibilities, and the time you can commit to working out. It's critical to be practical about what you can accomplish given your conditions. Setting a particular time period, for example, meaning to arrive at your objective in 90 days, makes a need to get moving and center.

Chapter 3

The Force of Activity: Developing Fortitude, Perseverance, and Adaptability

Key Thought 1

Choosing the Right Work-out Daily Practice for You

Choosing the right workout routine is fundamental for building a supportable and charming wellness practice. With innumerable choices accessible, finding a workout schedule that lines up with your objectives, inclinations, and actual capacities is critical to long-haul adherence and achievement. Consider the accompanying variables while picking the right work-out daily schedule for you:

Evaluate Your Objectives: Begin by explaining your wellness objectives. Would you like to work on cardiovascular well-being, develop fortitude and muscle, increment adaptability, get fitter, or upgrade in general prosperity? Distinguishing your objectives will assist you with zeroing in on the kinds of activities that best help them.

Think about Your Inclinations: Pick exercises that you truly appreciate. In the event that you disdain running, there's a compelling reason need to drive yourself to turn into a sprinter. Search for exercises that you see as tomfoolery, connecting with, and pleasant. It very well may be moving, swimming, cycling, climbing, combative techniques, group activities, or gathering wellness classes. At the point when you partake in the action, you're bound to stay with it.

Survey Your Actual Capacities: Consider your ongoing wellness level, any well-being concerns, or actual limits you might have. On the off chance that you're new to practice or have explicit contemplations, talking with medical services proficient or ensured wellness master can assist you with picking practices that are protected and suitable for your body.

Balance Cardiovascular, Strength, and Adaptability Preparing: A balanced workout routine commonly incorporates components of cardiovascular activity, strength preparation, and adaptability work. Cardiovascular activity, like energetic strolling, running, cycling, or swimming, further develops heart well-being and perseverance. Strength preparing works out, utilizing loads or opposition, assists with developing muscle fortitude and bone thickness. Adaptability works out, like yoga or extending, advances joint portability and diminishes the gamble of wounds. Find the right equilibrium of these parts in view of your objectives and interests.

Stir It Up: Assortment is vital to staying away from fatigue and forestalling leveling. Consolidating a blend of various exercises keeps your exercises fascinating as well as difficulties your body in various ways. You can shift back and forth between high-impact exercises, strength instructional courses, and adaptability-centered meetings consistently. Explore different avenues regarding various classes, activities, or sports to keep your routine new and energizing.

Key 2

Cardiovascular Exercises: Helping Your Heart Wellbeing

Taking part in ordinary cardiovascular exercises is a superb method for further developing your heart's well-being and in general cardiovascular wellness. These exercises hoist your pulse, increment your bloodstream, and reinforce your heart and lungs. Integrating cardiovascular activities into your wellness routine offers various advantages, like decreasing the gamble of coronary illness, further developing perseverance, overseeing weight, and upgrading general prosperity. Here are a few powerful cardiovascular exercises to support your heart's well-being:

Energetic Strolling: Strolling is a low-influence and open cardiovascular activity reasonable for all wellness levels. Integrate lively strolling into your day-to-day daily practice by going for longer strolls, expanding your speed, and looking for uneven landscapes. Go for the gold 30 minutes of lively strolling most days of the week.

Running or Running: Running or running is a high-influence cardiovascular activity that can essentially hoist your pulse. Begin step by step on the off chance that you're a fledgling and bit by bit increment your running time and power. Put forth reachable objectives, like running a specific distance or working on your speed over the long haul.

Cycling: Cycling is a flexible cardiovascular activity that can be performed outside or inside on an exercise bike. It reinforces your leg muscles, works on cardiovascular perseverance, and is delicate on the joints. You can cycle on streets, and trails, or use exercise bikes at the rec center or home.

Swimming: Swimming is a low-influence, full-body exercise that gives fantastic cardiovascular advantages. It works your heart and lungs while additionally captivating your muscles. Whether you swim laps, take part in water heart-stimulating exercise, or essentially appreciate sporting swimming, the water offers obstruction and works on cardiovascular wellness.

Stop-and-go aerobic exercise (HIIT): HIIT exercises include short eruptions of extreme activity followed by brief recuperation periods. These exercises are profoundly productive and powerful for cardiovascular wellness. They can be performed with different activities, for example, running, hopping jacks, or burpees. HIIT meetings are typically more limited in length however require the greatest exertion.

Bunch Wellness Classes: Joining a bunch of wellness classes like vigorous exercise, Zumba, dance cardio, kickboxing, or indoor cycling can make cardiovascular exercises more pleasant and social. These classes frequently integrate music, movement, and energetic teachers, making a tomfoolery and inspiring environment.

Aerobics: High-intensity exercise joins cardiovascular activity with strength preparation. It includes playing out a progression of activities focusing on various muscle bunches with negligible in the middle between. This exercise keeps your pulse raised while additionally developing fortitude and perseverance.

Working out with Rope: Bouncing rope is a straightforward yet compelling cardiovascular activity that should be possible in practically any place. It consumes calories, further develops coordination, and fortifies your cardiovascular framework. Begin with more limited stretches and continuously increment your skipping time

Key thought 3

Strength Preparation: Chiseling Your Muscles and Bones

Strength preparing, otherwise called opposition preparing or weightlifting, is a strong type of activity that spotlights working on solid strength, perseverance, and tone. While it very well might be ordinarily connected with building muscle, strength preparation offers various advantages past feel. It shapes your muscles, fortifies your bones, further develops digestion, upgrades athletic execution, and advances generally practical wellness. This is the way you can integrate strength preparation into your wellness schedule:

Grasp the Nuts and bolts: Strength preparation includes applying for protection from your muscles, which should be possible by utilizing different hardware like free weights, hand weights, obstruction groups, or weight machines. It's essential to learn appropriate structure and procedure to boost results and limit the gamble of injury. Consider working with a certified strength and molding subject matter expert or fitness coach to first aid you.

Begin with Compound Activities: Compound activities draw in various muscle bunches at the same time, making them profoundly productive and successful. These activities incorporate squats, deadlifts, seat presses, jumps, and pull-ups. Compound activities invigorate muscle development, increment by and large strength, and give a practical development design that converts into everyday exercises.

Progress Bit by bit: Start with lighter loads or obstruction and continuously increment the force as your solidarity moves along. This ever-evolving over-burden rule difficulties your muscles, permitting them to adjust and develop further after some time. Continuous movement forestalls wounds and guarantees consistent advancement.

Incorporate Disengagement Activities: Seclusion practices target explicit muscle gatherings and assist with refining muscle definition and balance. Models incorporate bicep twists, rear arm muscle augmentations, calf raises, and sidelong raises.

These activities can be consolidated close by compound developments or used to target explicit regions you wish to zero in on.

Fluctuate Reiterations and Sets: To foster strength and muscle perseverance, change the number of redundancies (reps) and sets you to perform. Higher redundancies with lighter loads center around solid perseverance, while fewer reiterations with heavier loads underscore strength improvement. A normal rule is 8-12 reps for muscle hypertrophy (development) and 3-5 sets for every activity.

Rest and Recuperation: Permit sufficient rest among sets and instructional meetings. Your muscles need time to fix and develop further. Go for the gold 48 hours of recuperation time for each muscle bunch prior to preparing them once more. This might fluctuate relying upon your singular wellness level and power of exercises.

Focus on Appropriate Structure: Spotlight on keeping up with legitimate structure all through each activity to guarantee security and viability. Legitimate structure boosts muscle commitment and limits the burden on joints and connective tissues.

On the off chance that you're uncertain about legitimate strategy, look for direction from wellness proficient.

Balance Your Daily schedule: Join strength preparing practices that target different muscle bunches for fair everyday practice. Incorporate activities for significant muscle gatherings like legs, chest, back, shoulders, arms, and center. Expect to work for each muscle bunch no less than two times per week.

Keep tabs on Your Development: Keep a preparation log to record your activities, loads, and reiterations. Keeping tabs on your development permits you to screen your upgrades, put forth objectives, and make acclimations to your everyday practice depending on the situation. It's satisfying to perceive how far you've come and remain propelled on your wellness process.

Stand by listening to Your Body: Focus on your body's signs and change your preparation as needs be. In the event that you experience torment or uneasiness, counsel medical care proficient to guarantee legitimate conclusion and direction.

Recollect that strength preparing is for everybody, paying little mind to progress in years or orientation. It offers advantages like expanded bone thickness, further developed act, improved digestion, and injury anticipation. Whether you incline toward free loads, bodyweight activities, or opposition machines, integrating strength preparation into your wellness routine will assist you with chiseling your muscles, helping your certainty, and backing long-haul wellbeing and utilitarian wellness. **Separate It**: Assuming your definitive objective feels overpowering, separate it into more modest, more reasonable achievements. By zeroing in on more modest accomplishments en route, you can keep up with inspiration and praise your advancement. For instance, assuming you want to shed 20 pounds, set more modest achievements of 5-pound increases.

Be Adaptable: Perceive that progress may not generally be direct, and misfortunes or levels can happen. Embrace the excursion and be available to change your objectives depending on the situation. Adjust to changing conditions and pay attention to your body. Recollect that consistency and long-haul propensities are a higher priority than accomplishing quick outcomes.

Put forth Execution-Based Objectives: Think about concentrating instead of exclusively on appearance or numbers on a scale. Execution-based objectives, for example, expanding the weight you can lift or running a specific distance ceaselessly, can upgrade inspiration and give a feeling of achievement past style.

Record Them On paper and Track Progress: Report your focusing on yourself, you're helping your own life as well as setting a model for other people and making an expanding influence of prosperity locally.

Chapter 4

Fueling Your Body: Nourishment for Ideal Execution

Key thought 1

Smart Dietary Patterns: Part Control and Careful Eating

Creating brilliant dietary patterns is vital to keeping a reasonable eating regimen and advancing general well-being and prosperity. Two fundamental practices for careful eating are segment control and careful eating. These propensities can assist you with keeping a solid weight, forestalling gorging, and cultivating a positive relationship with food. How about we dig into these ideas:

Segment Control:

Know about segment sizes: Comprehend the suggested segment sizes for various nutritional categories. Use estimating cups, a food scale, or viewable prompts (e.g., a clenched hand for a serving of vegetables) to direct your part measures.

Peruse food marks: Focus on serving sizes and the number of servings per bundle while perusing food names. This data can help you comprehend and control your bits better.

Utilize more modest plates and bowls: Decide on more modest plates and bowls to make a deception of a more full plate. The research proposes that utilizing more modest dishware can assist with controlling part estimates and lessen gorging.

Be aware of calorie-thick food sources: Food sources high in calories or added sugars can sneak up suddenly concerning calories. Be aware of these food varieties and eat them with some restraint to keep a decent eating regimen.

Stand by listening to your body: Focus on your body's craving and completion signals. Eat until you feel contented, not excessively stuffed. It requires investment for your body to enroll completion, so eat gradually and enjoy reprieves during your feast to evaluate your satiety level.

Careful Eating:

Dial back and relish your food: Eat your dinners at a casual speed, biting your food completely and enjoying each nibble. This training permits you to partake in your food completely and advances better assimilation.

Connect with your faculties: Notice the varieties, scents, surfaces, and kinds of your food. Drawing in your faculties upgrades the eating experience and assists you with feeling more happy with your feasts.

Limit interruptions: Abstain from eating before screens or participating in diverting exercises while eating. All things considered, establish a quiet and careful eating climate, zeroing in exclusively on your feast.

Tune into your craving and totality: Check in with your yearning and completion levels previously, during, and after dinners. Eat when you are genuinely eager and quit eating when you feel easily full.

Develop appreciation: Pause for a minute to see the value in the food on your plate and the work that went into setting it up. Developing appreciation for your dinners can improve the delight and fulfillment you get from eating.

Key 2Healthy Eating on a Bustling Timetable: Feast Arranging and Preparing

Keeping a sound eating regimen can be testing, particularly when you have a bustling timetable.

Notwithstanding, with viable dinner arranging and preparing, you can focus on nutritious eating and save time and exertion during the week. Here are a few procedures for good dieting on a bustling timetable:

Key thought 3

Plan Your Feasts:

Put away an opportunity every week to design your feasts. Take a gander at your timetable and decide the number of dinners you need to get ready and which days you'll possess pretty much the energy for cooking.

Make a dinner plan that incorporates an equilibrium of macronutrients (starches, proteins, and fats) and various natural products, vegetables, entire grains, and lean proteins.

Consider group cooking: Get ready bigger amounts of food that can be utilized for different dinners over time. For instance, cook a major pot of stew or simmered vegetables that can be divided and utilized for snacks or suppers.

Make a Basic food item Rundown:

When your dinner plan is prepared, make a basic food item rundown of the fixings you'll require. Adhere to your rundown while shopping to keep away from superfluous buys and save time.

Decide on entire, natural food sources whenever the situation allows. These food varieties are normally more supplement thick and back a better eating regimen.

Prep Fixings Ahead of Time:

Commit a particular time, for example, an end of the week or a free day, to get ready fixings ahead of time. Wash and slash vegetables, cook grains, marinate proteins, and part out bites or smoothie fixings.

Preparing fixings somewhat early makes dinner readiness speedier and more effective during occupied work days.

Use Efficient Cooking Strategies:

Use efficient cooking strategies, like sluggish cookers, moment pots, or sheet dish feasts. These strategies demand insignificant active investment yet yield delightful and nutritious feasts.

Investigate fast and straightforward recipes that can be ready shortly or less. Search for one-pot dinners, pan-sears, mixed greens, or wraps that Part

chapter 5

Readiness for All Ages and Ways of life

Key thought 1 Fitness Tips for Occupied Experts

Keeping a wellness routine can be trying for occupied experts, yet focusing on active work is vital for general well-being and prosperity. Here are some wellness tips to assist with busying experts integrate practice into their bustling timetables:

Plan Your Exercises: Treat your exercises as significant arrangements and timetable them in your schedule. Shut out devoted time for working out, very much like you would for a gathering or arrangement. Adhere to your planned exercise meetings however much as could reasonably be expected.

Pick Effective Exercises: Select exercises that give the most extreme outcomes in a more limited measure of time. Extreme cardio exercise (HIIT), aerobics, or Tabata exercises are magnificent choices that can be finished in 20-30 minutes, yet still give a full-body exercise.

Integrate Exercise into Your Drive: If possible, consider dynamic driving choices like strolling or trekking to work. On the off chance that you utilize public transportation, get off a couple of stops prior and walk the remainder of the way. These little changes can amount to expanded actual work over time.

Enjoy Dynamic Reprieves: Rather than sitting in your work area during breaks, utilize that opportunity to move. Go for a short stroll, do some extended activities, or climb steps to get your body rolling and separate inactive periods.

Expand Mid-day Breaks: Use your mid-day break for active work. Consider taking a walk or tracking down a close by exercise center or wellness studio to fit in a fast exercise. On the off chance that time is restricted, even a 15-20 moment lively walk can be valuable.

Utilize Innovation: Exploit wellness applications, exercise recordings, or internet-preparing programs that permit you to practice whenever the timing is ideal. These assets can give directed exercises that should be possible whenever, anyplace, and frequently require insignificant or no hardware.

Focus on Consistency: It's smarter to take part in more limited gym routines reliably all through the week than to irregularly attempt to fit in one long exercise. Hold back nothing 150 minutes of moderate-power high-impact movement or 75 minutes of overwhelming force oxygen-consuming action each week, as suggested by wellbeing rules.

Include Others: Find an exercise pal or join a wellness class or gathering. Practicing with others can give responsibility, and inspiration, and make exercises more agreeable. Think about planning normal exercise meetings with a companion or partner to keep each other on target.

Make Little Way of Life Changes: Search for chances to be more dynamic over the course of the day. Use the stairwell rather than the lift, park farther away from your objective to get additional means, or have strolling gatherings as opposed to sitting in a meeting room.

Focus on Rest and Recuperation: Guarantee you're getting sufficient rest and permitting time for legitimate recuperation. Helpful rest and sufficient recuperation periods are fundamental for keeping up with energy levels, forestalling burnout, and advancing wellness execution.

Keep in mind, tracking down a harmony between work, individual life, and wellness is pivotal. Begin with little, reasonable advances and slowly expand upon them. Consistency and making wellness a non-debatable piece of your normal will assist you with making long-haul progress in integrating exercise into your bustling proficient life.

Key thought 2

wellness during pregnancy and post pregnancy

Remaining dynamic and keeping up with wellness during pregnancy and post-pregnancy is useful for both the mother and child. Notwithstanding, it's vital to move toward practice with alertness and observe rules intended for each stage. Here are a few contemplations for wellness during pregnancy and post-pregnancy:

During Pregnancy:

Talk with Your Medical Services Supplier: Prior to beginning or proceeding with any workout daily practice during pregnancy, talk with your medical services supplier. They can give customized counsel in view of your well-being, pregnancy stage, and any expected entanglements.

Pick Safe Exercises: Choose low-influence practices that are delicate on your joints and lessen the gamble of falls or stomach injury. Appropriate exercises incorporate strolling, swimming, fixed trekking, pre-birth yoga, and altered strength preparation works out.

Stand by listening to Your Body: Focus on how your body feels during exercise. Alter or stop any movement that causes torment, distress, or windedness. Keep away from exercises that include lying level on your back after the main trimester, as this can limit the bloodstream to the uterus.

Center around Center Fortifying: Participate in practices that reinforce your center muscles, for example, pelvic floor works out (Kegels) and delicate stomach works out. Reinforcing these muscles can uphold your changing body and possibly help in post-pregnancy recuperation.

Remain Hydrated and Abstain from Overheating: Drink a lot of water previously, during, and after exercise to remain hydrated. Try not to practice in hot and muggy conditions to forestall overheating.

Post pregnancy:

Observe Post pregnancy Recuperation Rules: Give your body time to mend after labor. Heed the direction of your medical care supplier in regards to when it's protected to continue to work out, as this can change contingent upon the sort of conveyance and individual conditions.

Begin Gradually: Start with delicate activities and bit by bit increment force and term as your body recuperates and gains strength. Strolling, post-pregnancy explicit yoga or Pilates, and delicate extending are great beginning stages.

Center around Center and Pelvic Floor Activities: Reinforcing the center and pelvic floor muscles is fundamental post-pregnancy. Begin with delicate pelvic floor activities and progress to further developed center activities, with direction from a medical care supplier or a post-pregnancy wellness-trained professional.

Key thought 3

Fitness for Youngsters and Adolescents: Imparting Solid Propensities Early

Ingraining solid propensities and advancing active work since the beginning is essential for kids and youngsters. Ordinary activity upholds actual advancement as well as adds to work on general well-being, mental prosperity, and scholastic execution. Here are a few critical contemplations for encouraging wellness and solid propensities in children and teenagers:

Empower Dynamic Play: Urge kids to participate in dynamic play, which can incorporate exercises like running, hopping, climbing, and playing sports. Give amazing open doors to outside play and cut off inactive screen time.

Show others how it's done: Be a positive good example by participating in normal actual work yourself. At the point when children see their folks or guardians focusing on exercise and driving a functioning way of life, they are bound to go with the same pattern.

Make It Fun: Spotlight on exercises that youngsters appreciate and see as tomfoolery. Integrate exercises, for example, bicycle rides, family strolls, moving, swimming, or playing dynamic games. The more charming the action, the more probable they will keep on taking part.

Support Cooperation in Sports: Acquaint kids with various games and proactive tasks, permitting them to investigate various choices and find exercises that they are enthusiastic about. Cooperation in group activities can assist with creating collaboration, discipline, and interactive abilities.

Put down certain boundaries on Screen Time: Support sound screen time propensities by drawing certain lines on television, PC, and computer game use. Urge children to offset stationary exercises with actual play and exercise.

Integrate Actual Work into Day-to-Day Schedules: Track down amazing chances to coordinate active work into everyday schedules. Urge strolling or trekking to school, using the stairwell rather than the lift, or doing family tasks together that include development and actual effort.

Advance Dynamic Transportation: Empower strolling, trekking, or hurrying to local objections as opposed to depending exclusively on vehicle transportation. This increments actual work as well as shows freedom and ecological mindfulness.

Give Various Exercises: Offer different proactive tasks to keep youngsters drawn in and forestall fatigue. Turn exercises, present new games or sports, and consider enlisting them in classes or local area programs that line up with their inclinations.

Underscore Wellbeing: Show kids the significance of security during proactive tasks. Teach them about wearing suitable defensive stuff, observing guidelines, and rehearsing great sportsmanship to forestall wounds.

Observe Accomplishments: Celebrate and recognize youngsters' accomplishments and endeavors in proactive tasks. Acclaim for their advancement, strength, and devotion to propel and build up a sure way of behaving.

Last summery

Fit Forever" is a sweeping aide intended to assist you with accepting a sound and dynamic way of life. This far-reaching asset gives important bits of knowledge and useful methods for focusing on your prosperity, characterizing and accomplishing practical wellness objectives, and picking the right workout schedules for your novel requirements. With an emphasis on balance, this guide stresses the significance of integrating cardiovascular exercises, strength preparation, and adaptability practices into your wellness schedule. It additionally digs into subjects, for example, evaluating your ongoing wellness level, defining feasible objectives, and the meaning of piece control and careful eating. Furthermore, "Fit Forever" offers direction on exploring wellness during pregnancy and post-pregnancy, imparting solid propensities in children and teenagers, and overseeing qualification for occupied experts. Whether you're a novice or trying to step up your wellness process, this guide outfits you with the information and devices to have a better, more dynamic existence.are not difficult to collect.

www.ingramcontent.com/pod-product-compliance
Lightning Source LLC
Chambersburg PA
CBHW070213260726
48658CB00006BA/2065